The S

Laura May

chipmunkapublishing
the mental health publisher

Published by
Chipmunkapublishing
PO Box 6872
Brentwood
Essex CM13 1ZT
United Kingdom

http://www.chipmunkapublishing.com

Chipmunkapublishing gratefully acknowledge the support of Arts Council England.

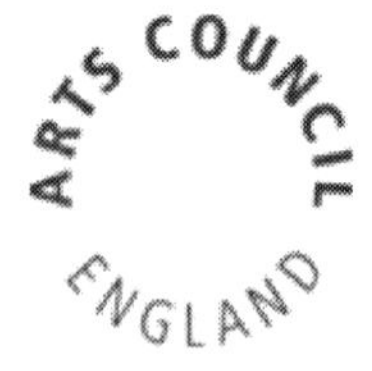

Dedication

For my Mum. I hope I can live up to you the way you have lived up to Nanny.

For my Dad. You have taught me so much, I will never forget that.

For all my family and friends – you know who you are, and I love you.

As always, for my angel, Brooke, who saves my life each day.

Acknowledgements

I would like to thank Chipmunka Publishing for allowing me to share my words, and special thanks to Jason and Paul for their patience and advice. Thanks to all my brothers and sisters, who are so close to my heart. Thanks to my parents, for giving me all the opportunities they never had. Thank you, sincerely, to Jay, who without which this collection would not have been born. Lastly, thank you to my wife, Brooke, for never 'handling' my illness and always knowing the words were inside, waiting to appear.

Author Biography

Born in 1983, Laura May is the oldest of six children, and always felt a bit 'different'. In 2008, after ten years of being treated for a range of mental health issues, Laura was diagnosed with Bipolar Disorder, and subsequently discovered she also has Borderline Personality Disorder.

Over the past eleven years, Laura has experienced suicide attempts, psychotic episodes and several bouts of extreme depression and mania, all of which she has tackled through her creative writing.

Laura May now works within mental health marketing, and possesses a degree in English Literature from the University of Hull. Laura lives in Essex with her wife and their 'babies', the many cats and dogs. Find out more about Laura May at www.lauramay.org

Contents

MIND

The Kitchen Table

The kitchen table,
in our home,
sees it all.

The kitchen table
is littered with my tears
where I have rested my head
on it's comforting wood.

The kitchen table,
in our home,
feels it all,

The kitchen table
bears the scars
of many red rings
from bottled nights gone by.

The kitchen table,
in our home,
hears it all.

The kitchen table
hears each letter
from the many witch doctors,
telling me my own mind.

The kitchen table,
in our home,
is where I fall each night,
with my love,
to talk about the day,
and forget tomorrow
is still going to arrive.

Clouds

Some days the skies are blue
and bright
without a cloud in the sky,
and your mind is clear
and the day slips through your hands like sand
and you smile easily.

Some days you wake
and the sky is cloudy,
the sky is so powerful in its greyness that you just can't see,
you can't think,
and you can't feel,
because you are empty

Your throat is thick with thoughts that won't form,
things you can't say,
as you struggle against the tide,
the waves that hit as you try to breathe,
try to smile.
But trying is not always enough to feed love.

Sometimes fighting,
even fighting dirty
with pills and words
and fear masquerading as love,
doesn't work.
You can't fight forever,
The clouds always bruise the sky.

My Mind

I wish I were writing of love,
Or hate or angry abandonment,
As then I'd be as passive as a child,
Watching the colours of this poem appear.

Instead I am writing of you,
As you pull me in with your skein,
With your standards slipping and your spite blatant,
You force these words

You push violently at my thoughts,
Tearing open each shutter,
And as they spill out onto this page,
I observe the forbidden, the loss of conscious,
Yet prevention is hopeless, dear pen.

Blank page, run,
Before the ink does,
Creating another poem filled with you,
Filled with the orange hue
Of another sunset in the park.

I am a Naked, Wild Colour

I am a naked, wild colour
like a splash, filtering,
I can be painted across any canvas.

I might be just too bright,
virginal before you,
I know sometimes I offer depth of vision that is too sweet,
I can taste it too.

I am an abandoned blue,
a roaring, lioness in red,
playing a game of chaos
with brush strokes on my skin.

My nakedness slaps you,
hits, hard, like honesty,
with colours from another age,
an age of want and need.

Smudge me, make me beautiful,
pull out the greys and blacks
from within my naked, wild hues,
and help me find the colour of my mind again.

Ruled Lines

Keep in the lines, keep it straight,
But I miss the violence of your kisses,
every present, everywhere, every line,
Blurs into treasured pearls,
Drums of rap-a-tap-tap

A witty remark breaks the beat,
To myself I tell this story, on ruled lines,
Like a ruled person, I bend and bow,
In the dark of my own pages.

Dust and ashes, my pages wilt,
Under the weight of lying lines,
Just don't steal my words sweet pen,
I declare, this drum is louder each night,

Rap-a-tap-tap they sing,
In my lungs, in my sight, wrapped around my tongue,
And the drums gain, gain, gain,
Lines that beat, at my feet.

Brittle

I wish I could tell you I was different then,
that I was happy, content, just a child,
but even in early budding years
I knew something was brittle.

I wish I could tell you it's because of divorce,
or a trauma, a scene, a fight in between,
but even in the first dawns of my days
it was nothing but my mind.

I wish I could tell you, blame it on the parents,
put it down to that event, let it soak in the past,
but there is no reason behind me
I just am this way, I am brittle,

I was brittle before my first tooth,
before my first gaping hole nightmare,
before the first, small innocent cuts of youth,
I was brittle even in the womb.

I tried to soften my mind, with fairy liquids and
powdered promises, dusty stained hopes,
But it was brittle before life threw itself at me,
so I am liable to fracture when submitted to stress.

Think

Never think,
I wish I could do just that,
Lying under too many stars,
Wishing for another name.

Say it's so,
Say thoughts may abandon me,
Say I'll never think,
Never think again.

Let the calm love me,
Cling to my skin,
Bury beneath this name,
Let the calm ease me.

Without thoughts,
Without these restless thoughts,
I might make another day,
Hold it in my hands.

Say it's so,
Say all thoughts are lost,
For if I never think,
I'll never lose.

Peace

The break, when it comes, it comes,
Too strong,
Soft against a mouth,
Too hard against a heart,

Moon hangs, accusing,
Behind me in the window,
And I can't reach peace,
although it stands there,
My hands, my useless hands.

This is all wrong,
Peace turned away from my reaching hands,
Useless hands,
That cannot hold on to sanity any more.

I beg her back,
Choke on my words, her name, this night,
My useless hands swallow my reach,
and this is all wrong again.

My Name

I am losing the fight,
against my mind,
unannounced, too quickly,
I forget my name,
and fall.

Slipping more and more,
I lose myself,
in the feel of just feeling,
in the touch of just touching,
and I fall.

So what do I want?
Just my name,
A name I can own,
Hold in the hollows,
and know it is true.

I am losing the good fight,
against myself,
trapped in senses, startled,
I forget again,
and fall too far.

And Poetry Found Me

And Poetry found me,
Curled in a doorway,
Awaiting my future.
Wrapped in the illusions of
A young girl.

My mind,
Consumed by the words
Of too many hazy images
And colourful hope,
Opened onto the pages
Of my future.

And in she stepped,
Forgotten thoughts released,
And screaming,
I met her in the farthest
Corner of each word.

And so I have escaped,
Taking her hand,
Into a world of
Clarity and contentment.

Symptoms

They say it's abnormally high,
this 'elevated' mood I love,
But I'm just dancing,
I'm just enjoying the thrill,

They say it's 'mania',
this love I feel for each moment,
But I'm just feeling, feeling
without thinking too much.

I know the low will come,
I know it will creep up on me,
A shadow to all my living colour,
But I don't care right now,

They say I'm 'euphoric',
Damn right I am,
I am a goddess
Creating the universe in my image.

I know the anxiety will soon join us,
me and my heavenly high,
But this hour, I shall pass it smiling,
For I feel just divine, doc.

My Other Half

You annoy me,
In the mornings,
When you smile,
And I want you, I want to be you.

When I say no,
You irritate,
Like a rash, you try to spread across
Each sensibility I possess,
And I sigh, Ok, I guess,

I would send you away
To the farthest, sweetest corner of my heart,
If only you'd stay there,
In the smallest room.

You don't listen,
When I try to fight you,
Knowing I'm using a pic'n'mix of cheap tricks,
Just to hold you down,

But I'm tangled up in you, me, myself,
I'm lost in this love of what I could be,
If only I didn't swallow,
If only I let you smile at me and win,
But you're eyes always make me fall, too easily,
they shine,

Against black tomorrows,
You shine, locked in this mansion of my body,
Telling no secrets if I hold the key,
My other half, my sins,
My angry, bright, shining girl.

Edit

I know I need to cut,
before I can even think about
the dissolve and the wipe,
but I can't.

I know I need to cut,
to keep the sequence normal,
to splice in the right place,
but I can't.

I know I need to cut,
to find direction,
to know my way,
but I can't.

I am just filming
the wrong moments,
I can't cut my life
where I want to.

Hey Baby

I stutter into the night, hey
Baby, hey
I let the rain in on my hair,
Look straight on
I say, just drive,
Just drive.

And the night flashes outside
my window,
Cities swallow me,
I say, keep driving,
Just drive.

I keep my silence, they keep their counsel,
The dark skies cry to me,
And I ask myself, can I let it go
Can I let go?

Fit the music around me,
The words,
I say just drive,
So I drive.

BODY

My Own Heroin

Give me pills, give me shots,
Give me everything you've got,
Give me highs so brilliant they blind me,
Give me scars from the lows that always find me,

I can take all the drugs, I know them well
They were there each time before when I fell.

Give me more to help me numb,
I know I'll always succumb,
although I fight and claw,
These wounds are too raw.

Give me something to swallow,
To fill up this deep hollow,
Make them pink, yellow or blue,
I don't care if they're true
I just need to feel whole,
As this day takes its toll.

Give me art, give me talk,
Give me therapy non-stop,
All the words in the world can't save me now,
To this terrible blackness I will always bow,

I bend, I break,
I take, take, take,
So give me pills, give me shots,
Give me everything you've got.

The Fully Divided Heart

I would love to tell you I'm different, I'm special,
but I cannot lie,
I have one too,
a fully divided heart.

I want to show you I'm unique,
But at the end of this dream,
when you cut open each chamber
you will only see one more fully divided heart.

My left lung, slightly smaller,
will seem identical to yours,
making room, as usual, for
just another fully divided heart.

Atrium, ventricle, valve,
whatever names you like to use,
will still apply to even me,
when you break my fully divided heart.

I want to say this black dog
makes me different, makes me superhuman,
I'd like to hold that distinction,
but I'm sorry to disappoint,
I'm just like you,
with a beating, broken, scarred
fully divided heart.

These Strong Hands

I try to control,
these strong hands,
which can paint so gently,
and steer so well,

I try to contain
each hazardous action,
but the stars, the moon,
have all been wiped out,

I try to build, instead,
with these strong hands,
instead of smashing it
all down again.

But on days like these,
when hands can't caress,
can't smooth, can't hold,
they are too strong.

Girl in the Bath

When I was nineteen, I killed a girl.
At first, I was slow,
I plied her with powder
and pretty, mixed cocktails,
and too many nights.

But she was tougher than she looked.
Each knock, she took,
Each fall, she bounced,
So I had to go further.

I filled the bath one evening,
knowing she wouldn't be able to resist
inviting warmth, bubbling scent.
I arranged my weapons
along the porcelain edges.

The water, when she sank,
was cooling at her toes, her nipples,
barely covered her fully,
yet it smelled so sweet.

The light bulb, swaying slightly,
with the movement below,
illuminated each vein, each scar,
each perfect imperfection.

My weapons were well chosen,
they did the job, almost,
startling the water with colour,
as if the water were white as snow.

Although planned, I plead
not guilty, for I knew not what I held,
as I raised my weapons high,

and pushed them down into her skin.

And so it was, at such a tender age,
that I killed a girl.
She only died for moments,
But I felt every one.

Two Legs, Two Arms

We have two legs each,
And two arms,
of course,
But as you know,
I have two faces.

Zeus forgot me,
his plan skipped my path,
and I will be forever
hiding behind my other face.

I am a single head,
I know, but inside
my other face defies
these two legs, two arms,

And promises a different future.
Fate brought us together
As Plato promised,
and now I am sewn on
to my other, ugly face.

I don't want to think of it
as my soul mate,
although it completes me,
for without it, I am nothing.

The Girl

Inside me, under years of practice,
there lives a girl I do not recognise,
she is made of light
so I hold her inside,
She might blind.

This girl, she breathes the rush,
she takes such delight
in a drink, in a fuck,
in the glorious chaos of night,

And though I tear across my chest
trying to keep her in,
some nights, and some bright days,
she escapes into my world,

She breaks my balance
uses my voice to scream, and giggle, and fights,
she takes my feet,
and She runs and runs.

Paper Thin

Another long day that I need to forget
Too many hours, time to pass, time to mar,
So I reach for old comfort, just to fight this regret,
With the reopening blossom of a friendly old scar.

The edges tear, so thin is my skin,
Like paper, I rip, I tear, I bleed,
I dig a little deeper just to get in
As this double-edged sword gives me just what I need.

I hate to love this so much,
But release, I'm afraid, is all I can see,
I hate to love this gentle steel touch,
But it is the only thing, right now, that will fill me.

Another long day I need to vanish,
So I kiss my wrists with a cool blade,
If I do this, I know, I might just manage,
As I press down I know the fear will fade.

So in love with the wrong world, I cry,
I know I'm stuck in this mud of the wrong time,
But my paper thin skin blooms and I fly,
And this moment, for now, is only mine.

Old Songs

Deep, old, broken songs
Sing in my head.
Not voices, not now,
just the torn lullabies of loss,

And I ache,
so much deeper than just under my skin,
I ache in my bones,
Bones I break too often.

These old songs, they haunt,
I can feel them in my mouth,
Hiding behind my tongue,
and they are breaking my heart.

Too many beautiful songs,
and I still can't find the words
To fight against these bruises,
To fight against these nights.

Rough, thick melodies
Circle my mind.
Not voices, thank god,
just the songs of forgotten souls,

And I ache,
so much more than this body can take,
I ache through my veins,
Lines I open too often.

The Shallows

Under the surface of the water,
I look up at the world,
Wishing to break through,
Longing to be someone else,

Within the shallows,
I drown in my cries,
I lose all direction,
I forget how to fly.

Under the oily cover,
I wish for more,
I long to reach up,
I hope against hope.

Within the shallows,
I suffocate in screams,
I swallow too much,
I forget how to breathe.

Under these shallows,
I am so lost,
Under these shallows,
I am a prisoner.

My River of Rage

Sweet seductress,
As our lips cry open,
Pain forgetting to lay silent
In the hollow of your bowels,
I hear you roar.

As you rage a spit,
Screaming against the banks of Nature,
You scare me,
My fear choking in salt,
And I am lost to you once again.

The day, as night,
Lays dark
Upon the shoulders of another hour,
As your selfish fit,
Pouring out against your scratched throat,
hisses in my ear.

I stand against your passion,
bold though bare,
and as the bruised air tries to escape you,
You catch hold of another howl,
And press forth.

Yet I can stand here,
Leaning over, trying to face you,
Who has so many faces,
As I know you'll calm.

And the lament of your agonies,
That you have touched and tasted,
Will cease to escape your blue lips,
And you will whisper again,

My River of Rage,
As the sky clears.

Breathe

Purple plastic, brittle against my skin,
I wonder how this silly little tool can ever get in,
But I push, and I pull,
And then I can breathe again.

I'm not always right, I'm not always clean,
But I try to stand tall and maintain each day,
By pushing, by pulling,
Just to keep breathing.

It's so small, so breakable,
Cold in my shaking hands,
But I know as I push and pull,
Another breath is rushing in to me.

If only I could breathe, deeply,
like everyone else,
I wouldn't need this plastic friend,
To push and pull the air into me.

Norma

Sexy mouth, ooh baby,
Take off that coat, the white hurts my eyes.
Don't you know I suffer,
As your back wins the audition,
And your eyes smile innocently.

Sexy mouth, ooh baby,
Say it ain't so,
Shimmy, shimmy away from the director,
Let that mouth pout,
Let it swallow your doubt.

Sexy mouth, ooh baby,
Don't you know I suffer,
When you sing those oohs and aahhs,
And brothers tear you apart inside,
And nobody realises how small you really are.

Sexy mouth, ooh baby,
I know that's not all you are,
But who I am to change legends,
To ask for a different ending?
I don't have your walk,
I doubt anyone ever could.

Too Blue

The sky was too blue,
the day I died.
Too blue, too innocent,
To look down on such a world as mine.

As the day stretched across it,
the sky was too blue
To hold all the secrets of my heart,
So I had to let them out.

The sky was too blue,
The day I spilled over,
The day I let go of it all,
Too blue to look down on me.

So it turned away,
and shone on another day,
Too blue to cast across me,
As I lay dying,
In my own skies.

Sweetest

As you fell,
And you felt and touched,
Conscious of your fall,
As I watched, breath bated,
As yours panicked

And then came the violent struggle
Of a deadening independence,
And you swallow,
And grasp,
For an air lost in love.

From beneath the surface
Of a suffocating water,
Your bruised lips become so kissable,
So appealing,
But my hands stay at my side

You're so ugly sexy,
As you sink,
Asphyxiated by this beating heart
That won't reach out to save you,
With its release

Your calm acceptance
Thrills me,
As I watch, waiting,
As you drown in me.
And it is the sweetest death.

HEART

Ribbons

Like ribbons of red, I feel as though
My heart,
My poor heart,
Is slashed and cut
Into thousands of beautiful
Ribbons of red

Can you hear me now?
Or am I lost in ribbons
In tatters.
I can hear the sigh of sorrow
In my heart.
My poor heart,
Bursting with the strings of too many violins, echoing
Repeating the cuts.

It's like a drug,
My sweet sorrow,
In my heart,
My poor heart.
It fills all my veins with the hum of violins,
The chant of ribbons falling into one another.
Am I lost?
Dear Lord.
I want you here tonight.
Allow me that. Hear.

Collide

Deep in my heart,
Beneath each layer of my skin,
We collide,
Like lovers should,
And I feel safe.

I am always floating,
Trying to grasp against the tide,
But you always steady me,
With touch and taste,
And I feel sure.

Without tomorrow, I slide,
Too deep under my darkness,
But you always present a day
Worth loving and living,
Your eyes,
And I feel.
More than I ever thought I could,
Like lovers should.

Mortar and Pestle

My wet heart
sits in this mortar,
chilled by its marble lips,
trapped in this bowl without walls.

It lies, unable to beat,
crushed under the weight
of a tired pestle,
that can't stop grinding.

The pharmacist tells me,
'Your flavour can only be found,
if we crush,
if we bash.'

I sigh, and let my heart
relent, cease, stop.
I know I will never be
Baba Yaga,
I will not fly.

The pharmacist, poor devil that he is,
can crush and bash forever,
But I know,
the muscle he grinds
was never meant to be mixed.

Duckling

Like an ugly duckling,
I wait for white feathers,
I long for the dawn,
and I sing the wrong song.

I am lost on a lake,
I see only my reflections,
Passing me as they go
Towards the right coloured down,

Allegedly uncommon, I am
rare, unique, but being rare
only makes me lonely
on this deepening water
that stares at the sky,

Like an old lullaby,
the water rocks beneath me,
but it doesn't hold me close,
Because I'm like the ugly duckling,

I don't belong, I don't bond
with this coarse world,
it tears at me like the bracken
edging this green water.

Just give me love,
give me a little love,
to whiten my feathers,
to help me spread my wings.

Lost Lover

I'm alone,
In this chair,
But I know you're moving
in the next room, shaded from the real me,

I leave before you wake,
I'm gone before
your eyes open, again,

But I want to stay,
In the hollows of your back,
In the cup, under your arm, of safety,
But I have to leave before I lose you.

I want to ask you
could you hold me?
Just until the noise stops?
Until I know I'm here?

Could you forget, just once,
that you've been inside me,
And instead,
Just hold me?

Just this once, let me hurt you,
Let me tear at skin and bones and us?
Can you make me feel,
Just this once?

But I will never ask,
I would lose you
before the words
finished forming,
I know this,

And you would join
the league of lost lovers,
Who pull at me each night,
In dreams I scream in.

The Luxuries

Sure, there are certain ones,
ones that seem so small,
that I still miss, even now.
A locked bathroom door.
Change in my purse.
Smooth legs.

Some I never cared for anyway,
Some I never notice now,
Even though they may be bigger.
Buying pills over the counter.
Judging others in a court.
Signing off on a loan.

Some I miss more than others.
A tall, cold Jack and coke
at the end of a long day,
A second, a third,
The indulgence of a bottle or two more.

I miss the thrill of
withdrawing it all,
Blowing roll after roll
On absolutely nothing at all,
Just having the cards.

But I have so many others now,
that I can hold in the palms of my hands,
knowing they won't cut me like shards of green glass.
I can wake without fear,
I can walk without stumbling,

I can be more, now, than I ever was before
when I was in the grip of a diagnosis,
I can taste the reality of the word

'Recovery', on my tongue,
so I would give them all up sooner,
If I could do it all again.

Charade

This charade is over,
but could I have my heart back now?
You're leaving, for now, so let me live,
Let me breathe again,
So I can keep you, my ghost,
away a little longer,

Stop haunting me, black, dog, cloud,
I smell you in this space,
But the charade is over, for now,
I need to fill my lungs
with purity,

I wish, more than anything, I knew
That you wouldn't return,
But it's never too late to call me back,
This heart never hangs up,
I need you, I know,
too much

I'm pushing, keeping you away,
For now, the charade whispers far enough,
But I taste blood, metallic, in my mouth,
And I realise my heart has burst
trying to let you back in.

Caught

Unlike you, I can't write down the words of my song,
I can't commit, in case they change,
In case they mould themselves around a new idea,
steer their course along the wrong lines.

I can hear my song, the sweet, sad strings,
I can feel the throb of lost promises in the notes,
but I can't find the words, they skip and dance
beyond my reach, always changing, changing.

I want to sing them, scream them,
find them hidden in my heart, beneath the bruises,
But I can never write them down,
although if I don't I know I will forget them,

Just like I have forgotten so many other songs,
I will forget my own as well, then I will be lost
to a wordless world that knows no direction,
I can't write down the words of my song now, or ever.

Assisted

Jim Jones said 'it's OK, go ahead',
but I know he was wrong.
He felt too little,
and knew too much.

I like to believe I did it
only for my own personal gain,
'gain what?', you may ask.
Only peace.

For my heart, long-ago torn
at the seams by
nights of bad dreams,
needed peace.

It was bleeding,
irreparable
so I fought with all I had,
just to find a little peace.

I never wanted my own
People's Temple,
or any assistance at all,
I promise.

My heart only wanted peace,
so I found it the only way I knew how,
and although I am selfish in my longing,
peace is all I can hope for now.

Undone

I'm undone,
Too far gone,
But heart says hold on,
And I try so hard to hold on.

To her. To me.
To the stars that burn,
To a heart that yearns.
Too far gone,
And I'm undone.

Push, wait
It takes my breath away,
And like a string I tighten,
against it all.

Hold on,
Til I'm gone
Lost on a whisper
like breath, I breathe,
And say, I'm undone.

Amica

Amica, amica, I will give you my soul,
you know no red lights,
as promised in the history,
but I love you all the same.

Amica, when you found it,
it was drowning in despair,
sewn together with raw stitches from others,
bleeding, open, ready.

Amica, you lifted it
to your sweet, red mouth
and gave breath to it again,
without taking anything in return.

Amica, you licked its stitches,
and put it in your hand for me
to take back,
so I took it back, my heart.

5/9

Turn it round,
Bring it back again,
Let's devour this shame,

Wrap me in this and you
So I'm not on my own,
They'll never have to know,
Let's take it slow

Let's make it into a bubble,
So they can't pierce,
I've been watching you for so long,
Wrapped in this shame of a secret.

There's this desire
Underneath, please let me in,
Under your bruises,
I wait to turn blue.

Change? Change?
I walk inside of another time,
I can't change,
no matter what I do.

Shadows of this sunshine,
I am here
Inside a thousand
unspoken sighs,

Sigh, let me crawl inside,
And make you mine
On the 5th, we collide,
and I know you feel me.

Foolish Devotion

Foolish Devotion,
Forget the master of your emotions,
She is lost.

Today, after days of building myself up again
You shattered me.
And all it took were a few words,
Foolish devotion.

No brandishing, forget teeth bared,
Just words,
And here I am, crumbling,
Into my red shoes.

Sparrow

She called me her Sparrow,
never knowing,
one day I might fly away.

She stroked my grey tail
with soft fingernails,
never knowing I might flee.

She called me her Sparrow,
thinking me tame,
never seeing the wild in me,

She hoped I would nest,
never believing
I would be called to draw any chariots.

She called me her Sparrow,
gave me the name thinking only
of my plump, brown shell.

She never imagined
His eye may be on me,
As I tumble down and fall.

She called me her Sparrow,
hoping beyond hope I might be,
always welcoming me back.

SOUL

The Great First Lines

I want to live in the great first lines,
I want to feel the power rush through me,
Go on, compare me to a summer's day,
Drink to me only with thine eyes,
I don't mind.

I want to bury myself in the great first lines,
I want to walk in beauty, like the night.
How do you love me? Go on, count the ways,
Come live with me and be my love,
I don't mind.

I want the great first lines written across my body,
I want my name wrote upon the sand,
I too, should like to rise and go,
For although the night is darkening round me,
I don't mind.

So many wondrous, great first lines,
which shall be mine?
Will I be caught in seasons of mist,
and mellow fruitlessness?
If so, I won't mind.

Will I be painted with a slash of blue,
or a sweep of grey?
Will I find my own scarlet patches along the way?
If so, I won't mind.

For I will have lived in the great first lines,
borrowed, maybe, but still all mine,
for I will breathe life into each note and line,
Until the stars burn out from ever gentle passing time.

Dear J

Sometimes, dear J,
I am ashamed of the things I have done,
I cower from the seconds I can see inside,
I feel reality slap my face.

Dear J,
some days are too long for me,
I can't rest my thoughts,
Everything costs too much.

These days, dear J,
I'm always behind on the rent,
I'm always losing my way,
I'm swallowing water by the gallon.

Dear J, I know
some things I hide from myself,
some details I obscure,
because they rush at me too fast,

But I'm trying, dear J,
to look closer at my palms,
to explore my restless finger tips,
to hold my hands steady.

Dearest, dearest J,
you have been a good friend
over these rough winds, these seas,
you have tasted my tears,

You have been so very dear to me, J,
you have held me anchored
through too many storms,
and I will thank you with stars one day.

Of a Hope

In this dirty hollow,
I smoke and write and think
And am content to merely breathe

And although I smoke,
And write,
And think,
Wherever I've walked out on,
You're much harder to hurt.

Like a name on the inside cover,
Your twists and turns burn into my mind,
As a thousand tales are told
From the lips of another night.

I could take a thousand pictures of you
And still never capture this moment,
This hunger, of a hope.

You don't ask for charity, or my gratitude,
Although you get both in abundance
And I am pathetically grateful for your indifference,
Though I can never walk away

In you I can never take off my watch,
And wander in your woe and love and crime,
Because I'd lose myself
In the beauty and love and grime

And when I leave,
I run,
Catching onto another blurred illusion
So that I don't look back,
Through the smears of dreams.

Nursery Rhyme

When I'm happy, I'm very, very happy,
I sing, I shout, I dance like nobody's watching,
I twirl round like a glitterball,
I am shiny, I am invincible,
I fly

When I'm happy, I'm very, very happy,
I am all I could ever be in the moment,
I soar above this cruel world,
and reach all the crying stars,
I fly.

When I'm happy, I'm very, very happy,
Or as it should be, 'very happy indeed',
Excitement pours, covers, shines,
I am Icarus, I am the sun,
I fly

When I'm happy, I'm very, very happy,
I am light, I am air,
I am beyond a care,
my fingers brush heaven,
I fly,

But when I'm sad,
I cut.

All I Can Carry

Hide my face, behind a cloak of insecurities,
And try to burn out these stars of mine,
Truth can never be discovered
If the stars are masked with Fate,

If illusion captures me
And holds on tight to stop the shouts.
Peace is a thing far from reach
And angels with black wings fly over me,

Build up these clear walls,
Let the dawns and dusks fade
Into too many moments of hazy recollection,
Just let happiness hit me like a bullet,

I beg, my bones beg, for relief,
For happiness I once held in my hands.
Finding no place in this castle of disbelief,
I can't carry it with me if I want to survive.

Let Me Make It

Sometimes I worry that I'm just not gonna make it,
Make it home, make it through the day
Make it mine, make it at all.

It hurts, when my body is ripped from the inside,
By the edges of these words,
And it scares me that I'll never climb out,
that I won't make it, I won't.

Another song, another strobe,
Pounds against me, each night,
And inside I am so ugly, I don't even feel it,
It would be so much easier not to wake up,

This idle brain is playing tricks on me,
Hoping I will curl into sleep,
Hoping I won't make it, won't care,
but I do care, let me make it, please.

Betrayal

Nature dances in my storm,
But my price, no doubt, is falling,
I am Lear, I am starved,
I reach only for the unreachable,

Half my care, half my duty,
I sing into the howling wind,
And know I can break all bounds,
In the darkened skies of oblivion,

A daughter of deception,
I betray, I betray,
All convention tears me asunder,
I have nothing, I am nothing,

Yet I fly, I soar, I peak above you all,
I am blind, as only the gods can be,
Reflecting the mistakes of man,
I am a mirror of betrayal.

In this play, I act out,
On a stage of destruction,
And everything springs from this,
The first scene, this sweet betrayal.

London Bridge

I can taste each slut,
The tramps, the muck,
Each alley filled with screams,
Each gutter filled with dreams,
And I am in love.

The forgotten youth,
The sordid filth,
Lying under my skin,
Edging its way in,
Lies also in my heart,
And I am in love.

From ashes to ashtray
I take this, another day,
And just under my tongue
I can feel it's begun,
Because I am in love.

My faith, no longer shattered
Picks up the pieces
Scattered,
Littering my love.

On my bridge, my heroine,
I wait for the day again,
Standing here,
Against the air,
In love.

The Lost Sonnet

My, what a sad hour is this;
When dark is cast upon the day,
And light is lost to other skies
And smiles waste, and seek decay.

Why should nightfall bring such ill
When day is bright and bold and true?
Night is no longer lit by the moon
But shadows lurk in grey and blue.

The sun retreats and hides away,
The black of night is clear and shown.
Sleep begins to replenish dreams
While in your bed you seek your own;

And so the night is all but lost;
In dreams that cause but only cost.

Catching

I keep catching myself,
A flash of colour,
A sharp scent,
then I am gone again.

I keep catching the day,
Warm texture of a coat,
Cold air in my lungs,
A deepening dark sky,
then it is gone again.

I keep catching a promise,
Of a happier morning,
Of a deeper knowledge,
And then that old ache resumes.

I keep catching clarity,
Thoughts pushing against me,
Knowing I will be OK,
then just another rush,
as emptiness returns.

I can't catch hold,
Of my dreams,
Of my hopes,
Of myself.

Inspiration

Let the grit in, under your fingernails,
Let the rain make you grey,
But when the lonely soul
Needs a hand,
Don't let the cold create shadows,
Or the heat be soaked up in your walls,
For his sake.

He knows he'll need you,
And you feast on his necessity,
Don't let the fellow fall
When he needs a word,
Or a colour on his canvas,
Or a simple note of light,
As the fall will be far.

Like all powerful friends,
You abuse each hopeful soul,
But don't let him cry out
In the darkness of another night,
When you can shed light,
You selfish thing.

Rot away, great beauty and art,
though remember your duty,
When the time comes,
The world will call on you,
To inspire her once again,
As you have each man of worth,
that hides in your attic.

Each Dream

You turn again, as the frost creeps in,
Into the room of sunlight
And the shadows seem warm,
Despite the chilled dawn,
And I wonder when it will be night

Your skin, although blue
Shows me nothing of you,
And I wonder how hot you can be
I try to be slow,
It's hard for me though,
When the rush is already in me

Can you see?
At my feet, you lie
And you moan and cry
At the harshness of day
As it's falling away,
Into a thousand sweet kisses
Of heat

And you turn again, walk right on in,
And in this room you'll stay,
Where each movement is light
Each expression is trite
And the night falls away from the day.

Settle on my Shoulders

Another day will settle on my shoulders tonight,
The sky still safe above me, another day lost to time,
Another day I have made it through, against the grain,
and although the sky is dark, sleep can't find me.

How can this day settle, envelop me, when I am not ready,
Not ready to soak myself in dreams,
not ready to cradle my head in hurt?
But settle it does, and my eyes seek the light
In the dark room, filled with my breathing.

Never great friends, sleep avoids me now,
As the day settles and slumbers against my thoughts,
Deserting me in my hour, this hour, of need,
All I need is sweet dreams, sleep, sleep.

But sleep will not settle like the day, so words will have to do,
I will have to wrap myself in tones and accept my losses,
for another day will settle on my shoulders tonight
whether I wish it or not.

Goodnight, B

Without me, you have everything
Sweet B,
you have laughter and life and love
all the 'L's that you need.

Without me, you have it all,
Sweet B,
you have tomorrow without fear
all the mornings you can feel.

So goodnight, B, sweet B,
I will dream of you,
beneath the waters of my sleep,
I will dream, only, of you.

Goodnight, sweetest B,
you have held on to me too long,
I am ready to sleep, dreaming only
of the angel of my heart.

Breinigsville, PA USA
08 March 2011

257247BV00001B/9/P